Table of Contents

1. Introduction...4
2. It All Starts in the
   Mind..7
3. Small Changes...................................10
4. Simplify It...16
5. Balanced Life....................................20
6. More Fluids.......................................22
7. Don't Forget about
   Fiber...25
8. Why Should You
   Care?..29
9. Conclusion.......................................32

1.

Introduction

I have been a registered and licensed dietitian since 2013. I have worked with patients in many areas including nursing homes, hospitals, dialysis centers and community centers. This means that I have educated young children all the way up to senior citizens on making healthier food choices.

Throughout the six years of being a dietitian, I have seen so much in the healthcare world with my patients and clients. In my experience, something in common that I found was that children and adults tend to have some of the same philosophies regarding food. They will chose anything that is greasy, salty, sweet, fried, etc. You get the picture. Mostly junk food or fast food. That's terrifying, considering that obesity is an epidemic in the United States. Not to mention other chronic illnesses such as diabetes, hypertension, hyperlipidemia, hypercholesterolemia and chronic kidney disease are all on the rise.

I wrote this book to motivate people to change their eating habits for the better. I eat a plant based diet and I would recommend that to anybody (especially if you are looking

Legal & Disclaimer

The information contained in this book and its contents is not designed to replace or take the place of any form of medical or professional advice; and is not meant to replace the need for independent medical, financial, legal or other professional advice or services, as may be required. The content and information in this book has been provided for educational and entertainment purposes only.

The content and information contained in this book has been compiled from sources deemed reliable, and it is accurate to the best of the Author's knowledge, information and belief. However, the Author cannot guarantee its accuracy and validity and cannot be held liable for any errors and/or omissions. Further, changes are periodically made to this book as and when needed. Where appropriate and/or necessary, you must consult a professional (including but not limited to your doctor, attorney, financial advisor or such other professional advisor) before using any of the suggested remedies, techniques, or information in this book.

Upon using the contents and information contained in this book, you agree to hold harmless the Author

Legal & Disclaimer

The information contained in this book and its contents is not designed to replace or take the place of any form of medical or professional advice; and is not meant to replace the need for independent medical, financial, legal or other professional advice or services, as may be required. The content and information in this book has been provided for educational and entertainment purposes only.

The content and information contained in this book has been compiled from sources deemed reliable, and it is accurate to the best of the Author's knowledge, information and belief. However, the Author cannot guarantee its accuracy and validity and cannot be held liable for any errors and/or omissions. Further, changes are periodically made to this book as and when needed. Where appropriate and/or necessary, you must consult a professional (including but not limited to your doctor, attorney, financial advisor or such other professional advisor) before using any of the suggested remedies, techniques, or information in this book.

Upon using the contents and information contained in this book, you agree to hold harmless the Author

to make health changes due to your decline in health status). This book merely teaches you to make small adjustments in your daily life in both physical activity as well as diet.

Don't misunderstand me, I do not eat healthy all the time. Dietitians are not perfect. Once in a while, I will reach for the comfort food or unhealthy food. We're human. It's all about finding a balance, with an emphasis on healthier eating patterns for better outcomes. It's about feeling good with the choices that you make every day, if you aren't already making them. It is also to reinforce what you may have already heard. Eating more healthy, natural and plant based food will improve your overall health.

Countless studies have shown a positive correlation between eating natural, plant based food and better overall or even improved health. This book is not just for you but also for your family, your children, your grandchildren and other loved ones.

Most people give up on their health goals before they even begin. Some people are looking to lose weight, others just simply would like to include more fresh fruits and vegetables.

No matter how big or small your goals are, know that you can achieve them. It's a process. If you are trying to eat healthier, don't think of it as going on a diet. It has a stigma attached to it. Even when you say it out loud or tell people. A better way to approach this would be to just think of it as a healthy lifestyle change. You want to change for longevity, to feel healthier, to be healthy and an overall better quality of life. You can use this book as a guide or better yet, as a reinforcement of advice you may have already heard.

2.

It all starts in the mind

I always wondered why people let their health deteriorate and how they got to that point in their life. I am referring to those who let their blood sugars get out of control or let their blood pressure skyrocket. If people only realized what a difference it makes to simply take care of their health, it would really change how they look at their quality of life. Preventative care is so important!

You may have heard the expression "Health is Wealth." It's true, your biggest wealth is your health. Your biggest investment is your health. Without good health, it is difficult to complete daily activities or do the things that you love. The sooner you start, the better it is and the easier it is. Genetics plays a role, that's true. Unfortunately we are not able to control our genetics such as what color eyes you have or if high blood pressure runs in your family.

You can only control your present circumstances such as the type of food you consume or how much physical activity you include in your daily routine. But why are so many people not able to do something as easy as including one serving of fruit per day or fifteen minutes of light physical activity? Why do some people already make excuses? Or even worse, they will make statements such as "I'll start tomorrow" or "I'll start next week." These phrases already set up your mindset for laziness and procrastination.

As I pondered this while completing my everyday activities of counseling and educating patients, I realized that most people give up on their health goals before they even begin. With any goal that you set out to accomplish, you first have to have the right mindset and the right attitude towards that goal. What that means is that you need to program your mind for success and do not even have failure as part of your vocabulary.

Materialist psychologists generally tend to agree that the mind is the function of the brain. What you feel, you bring about. You want to feel inspired and you should visualize your end result to motivate yourself to start off on the right foot. For example, if your goal is to lose weight, visualize yourself the size or the exact weight you would like to be. This stimulates your brain and you get excited about your new body. As silly as that may sound, it works. You are basically using positive thinking and the law of attraction to prepare yourself for your new body (if your goal is to lose weight that is).

Remember, this is a starting point NOT the end result. You also want to think or even speak out loud some positive affirmations. Examples would include "I am eating a healthy lunch today." Something along those lines. What this does, is that it sets up your mind and reaffirms that you are going to eat something healthy because you already expressed this out loud. Therefore your brain already received this signal and you programmed yourself for a healthy lunch. Again, these are just simple examples that you can start with.

If your goal is to get your body moving more, envision yourself walking or running around the park for ten minutes. The fact that you accomplished the goal that you set out (no matter how small) will give your brain positive reinforcement and therefore this will send a signal to your brain to want this feeling again. And the next day, you set out to accomplish that same goal so you can have that same feeling.

"Whether you think you can or you think you can't, you are right."

-Henry Ford

3.

Small Changes

Goal setting is very important when it comes to anything that you would like to accomplish in life. That can include dietary changes, physical activity and increased water intake. Let's start with a few examples. If your goal is to be healthier and live a more plant based lifestyle, you may be stressed out just even thinking about changing your diet overnight. Start with a small change in the right direction. When you have breakfast, swap your egg muffin sandwich for whole wheat toast with almond butter and sliced bananas. Try to do this every day for a week. You may want to switch up the different types of fruit or nut butters so you do not get tired of eating the same thing every morning. So instead of switching all of your meals at once, which may overwhelm you, start with just one meal--- switch your breakfast to a healthy alternative for a week.

The next week, start replacing your lunch to make it more plant based. So for example, swap your hamburger for rice with beans. Add some roasted or fresh vegetables to make your meal more colorful. This is the way that you should picture your meals. Is my meal colorful enough? You should try to "eat the rainbow" to be able to get a range of different vitamins and minerals. It gets easier to add just one more change (in this case changing your lunch) and this way you do not have too many changes all at once. You will not be overwhelmed and you will ease more into it.

It takes about twenty-one days to make or break a habit. That is why it is easy to program ourselves. It is actually harder to de-program ourselves, because you have to erase the negative thinking. With that in mind, just know that this is a process and you will learn what is best for yourself along the way.

If your goal is to also add more exercise (or your primary care physician advised you to do so) the same rules apply. The first week, try to walk for ten to fifteen minutes outside. Then the following week, try to walk for twenty to thirty minutes. Each week you add intervals of ten to fifteen minutes. You are building up and increasing your stamina. Your body releases endorphins, a neurochemical that boosts your mental health. Therefore, if it feels good when you are exercising and chances are you will repeat this activity.

You may have already heard of runner's high. That is a bit extreme, I am not advising you to start running miles and miles. But a runner's high is basically when you have a rush of endorphins; a state of euphoria. So when runner get to that stage, that's why they will run again the next day (or in a few days, depending on what your exercise routine is). Think of the mind body connection.

When most people set out to achieve a goal, they tend to focus only on the end result. That is a great start because it motivates you and gets you inspired. But you also need to have little celebrations along the way.

Let's use the example of the most common goal for most people which is to lose weight. If your goal is to lose fifty pounds in the next ten months, to a lot of people that would be considered a big goal. So if someone has lost only eight pounds in four months, he or she may get discouraged and simply will give up altogether. Instead of looking at the eight pound weight loss as an accomplishment, someone may view it as something negative and feel as though they are not losing weight fast enough. That's why it is important to feel good for any amount of weight you lose.

Again, this is just an example of a weight loss goal that someone sets out. Whatever you set your goal to be, celebrate the small milestones along the way.

It's a good idea to break down a big goal into smaller pieces. For example if you have a specific goal for the whole year, break it down month by month. Then take it a step further and break it down into weekly goals. This way you can measure your progress and adjust as needed. An example of this would be when people set out a New Year's resolution. Let's face it, for the majority of the population everyone's New Year's resolution is either to lose weight or work out more often--in general, these resolutions tend to be health related goals.

What happens during the first week of January or even the first couple of months of the year, people tend to be fired up for their goal. Adrenaline pumps through the body and everyone purchases a health club membership, if they don't already have one.

Generally, people will go to the gym on a regular basis and eat healthier throughout the day. But what happens toward spring time is that you see less and less people at the gym, it's almost as if they've given up or slowed down on their goals. Most often, this is due to people not seeing results fast enough. That is why it is better to break down yearly goals to monthly and take it a step further to break down monthly goals to weekly goals.

Here is an example to summarize small goal setting:

Let's say that your goal is to lose about 48 lbs. total for this year. (I chose 48 because it will be easier to divide and break it down when it comes to monthly and weekly goals). And let's assume you made this as your new year's resolution in January. Again, I am using weight goals as an example because it is easier to explain in mathematical terms and break it down to relate it back to goal setting.

-Yearly goal: 48 lbs.

- Take that and divide by 12 (since there are 12 months in a year). That equals 4 pounds per month. Break down the monthly goal into weekly goal, so divide by 4 since there are 4 weeks on average in a month. I realize that there are a total of 52 weeks per year, but in this exercise just to keep it simple we'll use 4 weeks per month as an average. So that will give you 1 pound of weight loss per week.

-Let's summarize the above paragraph:
- Yearly goal: 48 lbs.
- Monthly goal: 4 lbs.
- Weekly goal 1 lb.

Which of the above statements looks easier and doesn't make you cringe when you read it? Think about it. Losing 1 pound per week or even 4 pounds a month sounds like a more feasible goal than thinking of the total 48 pounds for the whole year. You have already set yourself up for success when you thing this way or when you break down your goals this way.

By reaffirming that it is an achievable goal, you are sending a signal to your brain as well as your subconscious that you will stick with this plan because you know that you can. We tend to process small information or smaller goals better because we can achieve them with more success rather than focusing on one big goal.

The recommended weight loss is about 1-2 lbs. per week. Anything greater than that may be dangerous. Always make sure you consult with your doctor or your healthcare provider if you are wanting to lose a significant amount of weight.

Goal setting is very important with anything that you want to accomplish in life, even health goals. We tend to put everything or everyone else before our own health. It's very important to take care of yourself and take care of your health.

4.

Simplify Your Goals

Do not try to complicate your goals. Make them as easy as possible. The thought of change scares most people. Let's face it, change can be scary. People are wired to stay in their comfort zones and repeat the same patterns over and over. As humans, it is easier to stay in the comfort zone rather than step into the unknown.

Let's pick a simple goal. If you are diagnosed with high blood pressure (hypertension), the first place you would want to start is to reduce your daily sodium content. Your doctor may or may not prescribe blood pressure medications depending on how elevated your blood pressure is. Following your doctor's orders with prescribed medications and changing your daily eating habits will have a good impact towards lowering your blood pressure.

A simple action step towards eating healthier would be to remove table salt from your meals, so basically not using the salt shaker. Instead, season your food to give it delicious flavor without the added salt. Then, incorporate more fruits and vegetables throughout your meals. A popular approach to reduce hypertension is the DASH diet (dietary approach to stop hypertension). The diet is very simple, basically what has been mentioned already. Eat more fresh fruits and vegetables, while simultaneously limiting dairy, saturated fats and most importantly salt intake.

Some people go overboard and think they have to cook fancy, over-the-top meals. You are only exhausting yourself and stressing yourself out. If you have time throughout your day and would like to experiment with different recipes, then that's awesome. Most people though work full time or even work multiple jobs and simply do not have the time to prepare these types of meals.

When it comes to snacking, do not reach for the chips or cookies. Grab a handful of almonds and an apple. Or peanut butter with apple slices. Keep it healthy and simple, since you are busy working or busy with other activities. It will save you a lot of time and effort if you just simplify your meals and snacks.

It is a smart idea to measure out portions, but only when it comes to the high calorie/high fat food such as nuts. Yes nuts are healthy, loaded with monounsaturated and polyunsaturated fatty acids. Keep in mind that it is still a fat, which means it will take your body longer to digest it and burn it off. You do not need to measure out your vegetables or fruits. Remember, you are trying to incorporate more of them into your diet. Fruits and vegetables are loaded with fiber, vitamins and minerals.

People will overestimate on what a quarter cup really looks like and fill up their whole fist with nuts as a snack. Yes, they are healthy because they provide protein as well as healthy fats. However, they are still a nutrient dense food. So grab a small handful using your five fingers and place the serving of nuts on the opposite hand. And that's it. Do not go back for seconds if this is only a snack. Again, they are packed with healthy oils that are essential, but if you are trying to lose weight these types of high fat snacks are the first thing you need to monitor as to how much you are taking in.

When I used to work in a community health center in New York with school age children, it was really surprising to see how many of them bought fast food right after school. When I would ask them why they bought unhealthy food everyday their responses were:

- "It tastes good"
- "It's easy
- "It's quick"
- "It's cheap"
- "It makes me feel good when I eat it"

These types of habits (along with many others) are the culprit of the rise in the national obesity epidemic. Just think how easily we can cut down on the statistics by teaching young children better eating habits. Children tend to mimic the world around them and they absorb everything around them like a sponge. So if they are surrounded by adults that make the same choices or watch television where they are being bombarded with commercials every 5 minutes about fast food joints, then that's all they know. You rarely every see a commercial about healthy grains, nuts, fruits, etc.—that's another topic too deep to dive into here.

In the above case, I advised the kids to ask their parents to prepare them a snack. I would give them an educational handout I made myself about healthy snacks, specifically after school snacks that can replace fast food. This is where I found out children make the unhealthiest choices. When adults aren't around and they can eat what they want and because some children ate lunch so early at school (as early as 10:45 am) by the time school was done, they were starving!

5.

Balanced Life

Everything in life is all about moderation and balance. You do not have to be extreme. It is okay to fall off the wagon every once in a while. You can have a "cheat day" and still jump back into action. Be flexible. Be willing to change, to grow and to learn. If your goal includes to eat healthy, home prepared meals everyday that's wonderful. If on a Saturday night you decide to eat out at your favorite restaurant with your loved ones, order your favorite "not-so-healthy" meal. Sometimes if you restrict yourself too much, then you end up going to an extreme.

If your goal includes exercising daily and you missed one day, it will not throw you off. Don't throw in the towel, per say, and just completely give up on your goal. Do not be so hard on yourself. Sometimes we tend to be our own worst critic. Shrug it off and start again the next day. Remember, balance! Do not get hung up on the guilt.

It may help to have an exercise buddy or even a group where you hold each other accountable or motivate one another. We all have those days when we just are not in the mood. Sometimes you get discouraged or feel lazy to get out of your comfortable home and go to the recreation center for physical activity. But when you have a workout buddy (or a workout group), you will be held accountable for showing up. A lot of the time people feel more responsible or obligated to show up to an exercise session because they want to prove to others (as well as themselves) that they can do it. The only person you have to impress is your own self. But it doesn't hurt to set a good example for others as well.

Another idea would be to join classes held at your local community center or gym. I have a coworker who will only exercise if it involves her attending a class held by an instructor. Otherwise, she will not work out on her own. There are actually a lot of people similar to her and can relate to her. That's perfectly fine. If you know that you may not stick to an exercise schedule on your own, it is completely acceptable to sign up for work out classes. Anything that will get you motivated and moving is great. I tend to work out alone because I like to be at my own pace. Find what works for you and stick with it.

6.

More Fluids

When making dietary or physical activity changes, most people forget about increasing their water or fluid intake in general. Our body is made up of about 55 to 65% water, so it is really important to constantly hydrate. Harsh winters and hot summers make us more dehydrated. The recommended amount of water is 8 cups (8 oz. each) per day or 64 ounces total.

Most adults barely can get in half of that amount. Why is water so important? Well, as mentioned earlier more than half of our body is water. After all, it is widely known that no human on this planet can survive more than three to four days without drinking water. It is essential to all humans as well as other living creatures and plants.

Water plays major functions in the body such as preventing constipation, lubricating joints, regulating your body temperature and much more. Keep in mind that water is lost through respiration and perspiration every single day. The average person loses about one liter (or roughly 32 oz.) of water daily through breathing and it is also lost through our skin. That is why there are many people today that are dehydrated or have constant dry skin because they barely replenish the amount of water what they indirectly lose.

Ideally, you should drink all of your recommended fluid as water. However, this isn't always the case. If you include juice, milk, tea, coffee, alcohol or other fluids that can also count as part of hydrating yourself. But be careful though because coffee, alcohol and most teas that contain caffeine, are actually natural diuretics. A diuretic will work on your kidneys by increasing the amount of water that is lost through urine. So in short, drinking more alcohol will actually increase the level of dehydration.

Drinking just plain water may be hard for some people since everything else we eat and drink has some type of flavor in it. The thought of having a plain taste may be repulsive to some people. I have heard from previous clients and that "Water doesn't taste good" or "Water doesn't taste like anything." which is why they use sweetened beverages. They have that good mouthfeel when sugar hits their receptors in their tongue. Water is not supposed to taste like anything, it is neutral.

There is a solution to drinking more water for those that have an open mind. You can try flavored water, and I'm sure most people have tried them already since they are everywhere!

There are so many different flavored water from many companies that you can't help but to try them. There are carbonated or flat flavored beverages.

You can even flavor your water on your own. Cut up a few slices of orange or lemon and place those slices in your cup of water. The flavor will seep in to the cup of water, flavoring it naturally. Along with flavor, there will also be vitamin C. The health benefits of vitamin C include being an antioxidant fighting off free radicals, as well as boosting your skin's collagen production. You can try it with other fruits as well such as cucumber, strawberry, lime, etc.

Start carrying a refillable water bottle with you at all times. Have one at your desk in your office or at your kitchen table, basically any place that will remind you to take a drink of water. Sometimes we get so caught up with work, family, stress, etc. that we forget to drink water. Some medications cause dry mouth, so don't forget to hydrate if you are taking any prescribed medications. If you need reminders, set alarms for yourself on your phone. As silly as that may sound, it works. Or even better, find a mobile app that has a reminder. I'm sure there is an app for that, there's an app for almost anything these days.

7.

Don't Forget About Fiber

Make increasing fiber intake as one of your health goals. We'll discuss why fiber is important in the next paragraph. Let's first take a look at the different types of fiber and explore them further. There are two types of fiber: soluble and insoluble fiber. Soluble fiber is found in oats, seeds, nuts, beans, lentils and other legumes. Insoluble fiber is found in vegetables and whole grains. The recommended daily amount is about 25 to 30 mg.

Try to achieve this goal from whole grains, fruits, vegetables, sees, nuts, etc. The typical American usually only gets about 15 gm of fiber per day. That's only half of the recommendation, which goes to show that we are focusing so much on protein that we forget about fiber.

Let's dive further into why fiber is important. Fiber is what keeps you regular, prevents diseases and helps move your digested food throughout your gastrointestinal tract.

So how do you include more fiber in your diet? If this is one of your goals, which in fact should be everyone's goal, you can start by just adding one serving of fruits or vegetables per day. Then slowly add more as the days and weeks go by. You always want to start off slow when adding fiber and increase it as you are able to tolerate it. Some people may experience some slight discomfort or bloating when first introducing good sources of fiber.

So in general, if you have not been including fiber on a regular basis, then your gut bacteria will have a bit of a harder time breaking the fiber down. Your gut bacteria will compile the proper enzymes to digest and break down fiber. This is because different fiber has different impact on the microbiota composition. You may feel discomfort and bloated if you try to introduce large amounts of fiber to your diet rapidly.

Most people don't realize that certain types of food which contain fiber, also are good sources of prebiotics. While everyone is busy trying to increase their probiotic intake, prebiotics are often forgotten. Probiotic are live bacteria that is found in fermented food, whereas prebiotics are fuel to help the good bacteria in your gut grow.

Maybe it's also because most people don't really understand why prebiotics are important. Prebiotic food increases the good bacteria that can boost your immune system. This is another reason to make high fiber food an essential part of your meals. Certain high fiber food contain prebiotic. Attempt to include at least 1-2 servings per day. Again, you want to start out slowly if you are not used to eating them. They are the following:

- garlic
- onion
- leeks
- banana
- asparagus
- artichokes
- lentils
- beans
- whole grains
- barley
- oats
- apples
- flaxseeds
- seaweed

As you can see, not only does fiber keep you regular but it also offers other nutrition benefits. When trying to include the good sources of prebiotics, it is more beneficial to eat them raw (for most of them anyway) since cooking will change the nutritional composition of food. Apples, flaxseeds and bananas are pretty easy to eat raw.

I cannot overemphasize enough how important it is to start eating good sources of both soluble and insoluble fiber. Your immune system will improve, you will become more regular (if you aren't already) and feel better overall. Fiber takes longer to digest because of the complex carbohydrates. In turn, it makes you feel fuller longer. You will not have blood sugar spikes, as you would with refined carbohydrates that contain little to no fiber (i.e. white rice, plain white bread).

8.

Why should you care?

I am sure at this point you are probably wondering why it even matters what you eat and why you should even bother to change your habits. Have you ever heard of the expression "You are what you eat?" If you eat legumes, nuts, fruits or any other food that comes from nature, you are taking in all the antioxidants, phytochemicals, vitamins and minerals that occur naturally in these products.

Whereas, if you reach for the junk food that is exactly what you are putting in your body (junk, chemicals, synthetic products, etc.). Think about it! There are ingredients that you are unable to even pronounce in packaged and processed food. If you do not know what these ingredients are and hence you cannot even pronounce them, why are you putting them in your body?

These additives and preservatives create more inflammation and stress on your body, because now your organs have to work overtime to remove them out of your system. Your body always tries to maintain homeostasis. So when you constantly feed your body unhealthy, processed food it will continue to work overtime and thus constantly be in a stressful, imbalance.

Often referred to as the "silent disease," chronic kidney disease affects about 14% of the population in the United States and that number continues to increase every year. I work in a hemodialysis center and I have also worked in a home dialysis center (which includes peritoneal dialysis and home hemodialysis). I am passionate about nutrition, especially when it comes to kidney disease because unfortunately there is not enough education towards preventative care. That is why I wrote this book and structured it in a way to make people aware of their health including diet, physical activity and positive mindset.

It is really a holistic approach. Of course I recommend people, especially those predisposed to kidney disease, to follow up with their nephrologist or primary care physician on a regular basis. This goes for any disease one is predisposed to: diabetes, heart disease, etc. This is also what I recommend to patients that I already have.

But it should not stop there. Complete your own research, take care of your body and mind. What is it that you need to do and that you can do right now. For example, if you have just been diagnosed with hypertension start by cutting down on your processed food intake or just simple stop using the salt shaker to salt every meal. Taking this step, will stabilize your blood pressure and you will have better control. By taking control of your blood pressure now, you will reduce your risk of kidney disease, kidney stones, etc.

In my years of work in healthcare, I found that a lot of people did not realize that one medical issue may lead to another. For example, I had a patient once cry that he had no idea that his uncontrolled hypertension over the years would lead to damaging his kidneys. Had he known, he would have taken better care of himself. Some people may take it lightly and think that nothing will occur from their uncontrolled high blood pressure. Sometimes that is the case. Not all people end up with kidney disease if they have a history of high blood pressure. But the chances are much greater.

Unfortunately, that's the case that happens most often. Most people are not educated enough on preventative care and so they put their health at risk later down. Part of it really has to do with educating yourself and really investing in your health.

9.

Conclusion

By now you have a well-rounded idea of how to be healthier in any aspect of your life. Regardless of what that may look like to you. Everyone has a different idea of healthy and what good health means to them. If it is to increase your physical activity, change your eating habits, increasing fiber or fluid intake, it all begins with a decision to change your lifestyle.

It can be overwhelming at first to make changes on your own. Having a support system is really helpful (such as your family or friends). Don't hesitate to reach out for professional help such as a dietitian or other healthcare professionals. It means that you are serious about accomplishing your goals and want to be on the right path. Even if it is for maintenance of good health that you may already have, it is still important.

For example if you are diabetic and have a referral by your primary care physician, Medicare part B will pay for medical nutrition therapy (MNT) to speak with a registered dietitian. So it is always good to just go in to make sure you are on the right track (even if you have controlled blood sugars). A dietitian may help you with any questions you have or if you wanted a weight loss plan, while being cautious of maintaining stable blood sugar. The goal is that you feel healthy, you feel good about yourself and continue a healthy lifestyle without feeling as if you are depriving yourself.

All in all, it starts with an idea or goal in your mind. You convince yourself that you can achieve it (because you can) and then you work on your goals with small changes at first. Including physical activity, more fluids, increasing your fiber intake with your end vision focused on being your own version of healthy. Celebrate along the way with any small accomplishments that are important to you, keeping in mind your end goal. So I definitely encourage you to take care of your health, your mind and set out to accomplish your goals!

Bibliography

McLeod, S. A. (2007). Mind body debate. Retrieved from https://www.simplypsychology.org/mindbodydebate.html

"Kidney Statistics for the United States." (2016). National Institute of Health. 2019. https://www.niddk.nih.gov/health-information/health-statistics/kidney-disease

"Fiber" The Nutrition Source. 2019. Harvard.edu https://www.hsph.harvard.edu/nutritionsource/carbohydrates/fiber/